Walk Off Weight With Your Pedometer

A Simple 28 Day Pedometer Walking Program

Jan Small

DISCLAIMER AND/OR LEGAL NOTICES

This publication provides information for general purposes only and is not intended as a substitute for medical or health advice from health care professionals.

The information within represents the views of the author at the date of publication and as such may be subject to change as new information comes to light.

The accuracy, completeness and suitability of the material for your particular needs has not been assessed or verified and cannot be guaranteed.

You bear responsibility for your own health research and decisions and must consult with a professional health care adviser before embarking on a weight loss or exercise program or making any personal health decisions.

No liability will be accepted for the use of any information contained within this publication or obtained by following links or recommendations within it. By reading this book, you assume all risks associated with using the advice given below, with a full understanding that you, solely, are responsible for anything that may occur as a result of putting this information into action in any way, and regardless of your interpretation of the advice.

Walk Off Weight With Your Pedometer

A Simple 28 Day Pedometer Walking Program

Jan Small

Table of Contents

Introduction

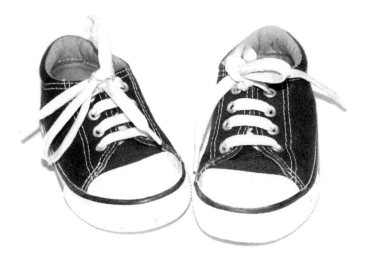

With this guide you have a simple method of losing weight and getting fitter in just 4 weeks without ever having to go to the gym or learn any new complicated techniques.

Read through the whole guide before you begin your program, check with your doctor that the Walk Off Weight With Your Pedometer plan is OK for you and then get walking!

Why walk?

You have made the right choice in deciding to walk –
here's why.

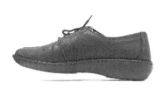 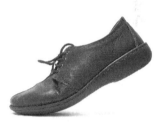

Walking Is Simple

Almost anyone without major physical restrictions can
walk and it's an exercise you can do your whole life long -
you can start no matter how old or how big you are.

Walking Has No Learning Curve

You don't need to learn any new techniques to get walking (although improving your posture using the guidelines
in the Plan is a good idea if you are going to walk a lot).

You Can Start Where You Are

Walking requires no particular level of fitness – you can
begin no matter how fit (or unfit) you are.

You Don't Need Special Equipment

If you have a comfortable pair of shoes you're good to go. Although we will be using a pedometer in our plan you can still walk with or without one. And pedometers are low in price and readily available.

You Don't Need to Go Anywhere

Walking can be done anywhere. You can start outside your front door and walk around the block

It's Convenient

Walking can be fitted into your life more easily than other forms of exercise. There's no need to get changed into exercise gear for a quick walk. You can walk at home or outside. You can spend 5 minutes walking or an hour.

It's Habit Forming

The more you walk, the better you'll feel and the more you'll want to walk. This helps you keep up your exercise program. Other forms of exercise are tougher, especially at the beginning and this can mean you give up before you really get going.

Walking Firms You Up

Walking helps tone your stomach muscles, hips, thighs and bottom. It works all the major muscles and helps strengthen them.

Walking Helps Your Circulatory System

Walking improves your circulation, helping distribute blood to every part of your body. It will boost your skin too.

Walking Is a Natural Anti-Depressant

Walking makes you feel better. It helps you sleep better, combat stress and depression and put problems in perspective.

Walking Does Not Put A Lot Of Stress On Your Joints

Walking gives you all the cardiovascular benefit of aerobic exercise without putting too much stress on your knees, hips and back – all the benefits of jogging, cycling and aerobics without the injuries.

Walking Reduces The Risk Of Disease

Walking helps lower your risk of heart disease, cancer and stroke and may reduce your blood pressure.

Walking Adds Variety To Any Exercise Program

You can vary your pace, distance, location, terrain, location and your walking companions to help keep things interesting!

Walking Keeps You Fit

Walk regularly and you'll maintain fitness for life!

And of course, it helps you lose weight

How Walking Helps You Lose Weight

The only way walking will not help you lose weight is if you don't do it!

If you keep going, walking will work for you.

Keep reminding yourself **why** you are following a walking program. Whenever you feel your motivation flagging come back to this section to give yourself a boost...

1. Walking burns calories

Walking burns as many calories as jogging over the same distance. If you walk around 4 mph you will be burning about 5 times as many calories than if you were sitting.

2. Walking improves your basal metabolic rate

Your basal metabolic rate is the number of calories you use just to stay alive. The fitter you are and the more muscle tissue you have, the more calories you burn even when you are sitting around doing nothing or sleeping. And walking improves both your fitness and the amount of lean muscle you have. You will actually change your body composition by walking.

3. Walking Burns Fat

If you walk aerobically (meaning a brisk walk that leaves you a bit breathless but still able to talk) for about 45 minutes you will burn around 300 calories and about 180 of them will be pure fat. Regular walking increases the action of fat-burning enzymes.

4. Walking Reduces Cravings

If you are unfit and unused to exercise, any sudden vigorous activity tends to result in energy being drawn from the body's blood sugar stores. This leads to cravings as that energy needs to be immediately replaced. With regular walking, body chemistry changes so that you tend to more easily extract energy from fat cells rather than sugar stores resulting in fewer cravings.

5. Walking Is The Easiest Form Of Exercise

Most people give up on exercise because it's just too much effort to keep it up. But walking is easier to fit into your life because you don't need to get to a gym to do it or get changed into special clothes or get showered afterwards. You can fit it into the busiest lifestyle. It's easier to go for a walk than a jog if you're not used to exercise – therefore you're more likely to do it

6. Walking Can Be Stop-Start

You also don't need to reserve huge blocks of time to go for a walk. Walking can be a stop-start activity. There's no "all or nothing" with a pedometer walking program. Every step counts. With other exercise options you either get to the gym or you don't. You either go for a swim or you don't. If you know you are not going to manage to go for a long walk you can make up a lot of ground by simply moving more during the course of your normal day.

7. Walking Maintains Your Weight After You Lose It

Walking is one of the best ways to maintain your weight without having to go hungry. If you follow this program conscientiously you will feel so many benefits that walking will become an enjoyable habit you won't want to give up. After you lose weight, regular walking will ensure the weight stays off.

Why The Walk Off Weight Program Works

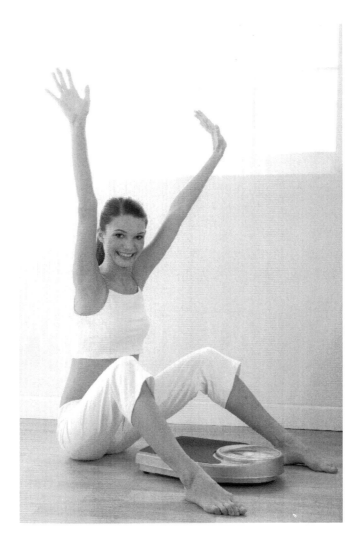

The Walk Off Weight program uses a particular approach to losing weight which means...

You Are Making Small Changes

In this program, you are making small changes rather than going for a big upheaval turning your life upside down.

Gradual changes to your eating and exercise habits are the ones which stick as permanent changes while those "change your lifestyle overnight" programs rarely last more than a week (no – you are not especially weak-willed because you can't keep to your strict program – believe me, no one does!)

You Will Feel Good Right Away

You know how it is when you come back from a vigorous exercise session after not doing anything for a while. You feel SORE (and worse - the next day you can hardly move). Not so with this program. You will feel invigorated and bouncing with energy and ready for more each day.

You Will Steadily Lose Weight

With this program. it won't be a case of losing 4 pounds in one week, 2 pounds the next and putting it all back on over the following 2 weeks. Be ready for less spectacular weight loss in the beginning – we are aiming for the kind of weight loss which stays off permanently – a steady 1 to 2 lbs weight loss week after week. But that 1 to 2lbs a week grows into a spectacular weight loss while your friends who lost so much weight in the beginning are licking their wounds and wondering where they went wrong.

You Will Be Healthier And Fitter As Well As Slimmer

Because you are exercising to lose weight and losing weight gradually you will improve your general health and maintain your muscle and skin tone.

Many diets which promote rapid weight loss mean losing muscle tissue as well as fat and lead to sagging skin and rapid regain of lost weight. You will not only lose weight but also look better better and feel better on this program.

Why Use a Pedometer?

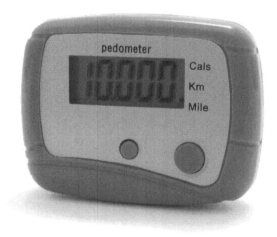

They say that what gets measured gets done. And a pedometer is a fun way of measuring how much exercise you get each day. Even if you think you had an active day the pedometer might just tell you something else :) Sometimes we think we are active when we are merely stressed out or busy.

By challenging yourself to a certain number of steps every day and making every step count, you will find yourself moving more than you otherwise would.

Research has shown that the difference between those who put on weight and those lucky people who stay slender is often due to normal activity levels.

It is more to do with how much they move about in every-day life than how much formal exercise they take or how much they eat.

Slender people move an average of 350 calories a day more as they go about their lives. That's an extra pound of fat's worth of calories they use every 10 days without taking any formal exercise at all!

If you wear your pedometer all the time, it will help you join that lucky group by encouraging you to move more as you go about your normal day.

The beneficial results are backed up by scientific research. For example, The Journal of the American Medical Association published the results of a study in Nov. 2007 concluding that, "the use of a pedometer is associated with significant increases in physical activity and significant decreases in body mass index and blood pressure."

How A Pedometer Works

What may seem like a complicated scientific instrument to detect the fact that you have taken a step is actually very simple.

A pedometer contains a sensor which detects movement from your hips (by detecting a change to your center of gravity) and each movement is counted as a step.

When you program a pedometer with your average stride length (see the "How to Use a Pedometer" section), it can also determine the approximate distance you travel.

How to Choose a Pedometer

Don't worry if you have already bought a pedometer –
you'll get on just fine **as long as you use it!** If you have
yet to buy one, here are the things to think about...

1. Type of mechanism

The sensor in your pedometer can be one of three types
of mechanism.

The most accurate is a piezoelectric accelerometer type
mechanism found in more expensive pedometers. This is
followed in accuracy by a coiled-spring type mechanism
and lastly and least accurate a hairspring mechanism.

With the least accurate cheapest pedometers you are
likely to find steps being counted when you are not making any (such as when you bend to tie your shoes) and
steps not being counted when you are (although this is
more likely to be caused by not wearing the pedometer
correctly).

If you have yet to buy your pedometer it is worth paying a
little more for a digital model which is least likely to count
"false steps" rather than expecting something which cost
a couple of pounds to be an accurate scientific instrument.

If you have (or want to buy) a cheaper one and really
want to get an accurate picture you could spend a little

time determining the average count on your pedometer over several sets of 100 steps (counted manually).

Then you can factor in how inaccurate your model is from then on when monitoring your steps. For example, if your pedometer, clocks up 105 steps on average for every 100 actual steps, you can reduce your totals each day accordingly.

On the other hand, unless that sort of thing bugs you, don't get caught up in worrying about exact steps. It is really not going to matter too much in the scheme of things. We are looking at an order of magnitude here – and building up the number of steps day by day is more important than complete accuracy.

2. Features

Your pedometer may have features other than counting your steps if you choose a more expensive model.

Some have calorie counters showing how many calories you are burning as you walk. While these are not particularly accurate, especially in the cheapest models, they may serve as a bit of motivation!

Some measure distance as well as steps – and this is a good motivational feature too (although there are other ways of measuring distance).

More sophisticated models may come with a built in radio or compass, while some pedometers are themselves just additional features on a mobile phone or MP3 player.

Just think about what you will actually use before you pay for a lot of features you don't need.

It's better to spend money on a more accurate basic pedometer than on gimmicks.

3. Price

Of course your budget may be the overriding factor in your choice. I have seen pedometers as cheap as a cup of coffee and of course, there's no limit when you're talking about multi-functional gadgets but try and strike a balance between quality, features and price so that you get something that you will be happy with.

Recommended Pedometers

If you're confused about pedometers a short list of re-commended pedometers may help.

As pedometer models change a lot, I have created a page on the web at http://walkoffweight.org with a selection of the latest recommended pedometers. All of these have great user reviews so you can choose one with some confidence that it will work well.

How to Use a Pedometer

If your pedometer is just a basic step counter and you are not interested in measuring how much distance you cover with your walking, move on to the "How to Wear your Pedometer" section.

However if your pedometer measures distance, you will need to calibrate it so that it takes the average length of your stride into account.

Your pedometer should come with instructions on how to do this but, if not, you can use one of the following methods.

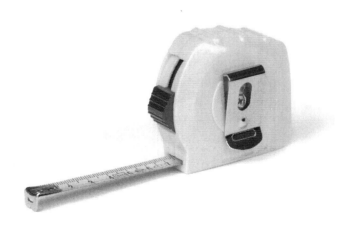

1. Measure 10 steps Method

With this method you take 10 normal steps on a flat even surface making a mark behind your heel where you begin and one behind your leading heel where you end. Then you measure the distance between the two marks and divide it by 10. That is your average stride length.

Although this is the easiest method, there is a problem with it in that you are measuring from a standing start which is not how you would normally walk over a longer distance. To get a more accurate picture use the following method.

2. Count the Steps Method

With this method you use a pre-measured distance of about 20 feet or 10 metres and simply count how many steps you take to cover it.

Start outside your pre-measured area so that you are walking normally by the time you reach the start line.

Then you divide the pre-measured distance by the number of steps you took to cover it to get your stride length.

Note that pedometers are best for measuring distance on flat and gently sloping gradients. If you are going up and down hills your stride is likely to vary a great deal and therefore average stride length will be inaccurate in those circumstances.

If you want to lose weight I advise that you walk wherever you like (hills are great), count those steps and don't worry about distance.

Measuring Distance covered without Your Pedometer

If your pedometer does not compute distance for you, then you can use the above tests to measure your average stride and then simply multiply your average stride by your steps covered each day, or each walk.

Alternatively, if you are walking outside there are some great online and mobile utilities Like Map My Fitness and Map My Walk where you plot your path on a map and it shows you the distance you travelled on your walk.

How to Wear Your Pedometer

Your pedometer will probably come with instructions on how to use it. If not these guidelines should help for most models.

Clip your pedometer to your belt or waistband about 5 to 15cm to either side of your belly button – this should be about in line with your knee.

Women may need to wear their pedometer clipped to their underpants if wearing a dress without a belt. (It may also work clipped to the centre of a bra – anywhere where changes to centre of gravity can be detected will work.)

Make sure your pedometer is straight and close to your body.

If you have a large stomach, try wearing the pedometer on your hip.

Some of the high end pedometers work even if they are kept in your pocket or bag as you walk. Check the instructions, if you have one of these so you know where best to carry it.

If you don't like wearing a pedometer clipped to your waistband, you will find paying a bit extra for one of these pedometers is well worth it. This is the kind of model I have and I find it is so much easier just carrying the pedometer in my pocket.

How to Check Your Pedometer is Working Properly

It's pretty annoying to walk about all day only to find your pedometer has only clocked up a few hundred steps so always check any new pedometer for accuracy.

Wear your pedometer and manually count while you take 100 steps then check how many steps your pedometer has registered.

Don't worry about a few steps either way but if you are more than 5 or so out then try re-positioning your pedometer until you get a place where it properly registers changes to your centre of gravity.

This may be the time to buy a new pedometer if you find that you can't get a result that is anywhere near accurate with yours.

When to Wear Your Pedometer

For best results for weight loss (and motivation!) wear your pedometer all day, as soon as you get up. I found putting my pedometer in my dressing gown pocket helped me to remember to use it!

Of course, you will need to remove your pedometer when you take your shower or bath and for swimming. (I haven't found a completely waterproof one yet though mine still seemed to work OK after I managed to drop it in a bucket of water – I did get it out and dry it off fast though!).

Register your results when you take your pedometer off to go to bed at night and give yourself a pat on the back for the steps you clocked up.

Before you Begin Your Pedometer Weight Loss Program

1. Check with your Doctor

Walking is suitable for most people but check with your doctor if there's any doubt about your health.

2. Find a comfortable pair of shoes

To start with any comfortable shoe will do but once you get the walking bug it's best to go for proper walking shoes.

Running shoes are not ideal (but you could go for these if you think you'll probably take to jogging later). These shoes tend to be inflexible as they have thick soles to absorb the shock as your heel strikes the ground so they impede the proper walking heel to toe foot movement a little.

There are shoes meant for hiking in rough terrain and hill walking but check that these are not too rigid for everyday walking. You may want to get different shoes for different purposes.

For normal walking look for:-

Flexible Soles

Choose flexible soles which bend in the area of the ball of your foot where your foot bends rather than at the arch

Cushioned heels

This helps alleviate any pain where the heel strikes the ground.

Room For Expansion

Shoes need plenty of room for your toes as walking for an hour can cause your foot size to increase temporarily by half a size. Look for a shoe with about half an inch (1.5cm) between your longest toe and the end of the shoe. Note that suitable walking shoes may a different size (usually larger) than your normal shoes.

Quality Materials

Choose shoes which are made of light and breathable materials such as leather or breathable synthetic materials.

Gender Specific

Buy shoes which are specifically made for women or men – women's shoes tend to be lower or v-shaped at the back as Achilles tendons are exposed at a lower level than on a man's foot.

If you're not sure what to buy get fitted by a specialist sports shoe store – not the ones where teenagers stand around looking too bored to serve you.

Some of the specialist stores have a treadmill and video set up where the store assistant monitors your movement to help select the right shoes for you. Buy from one of these stores if you can.

The 500 Mile Rule

Shoes need replacing every 500 miles – or when they have lost their springiness or padding. At the moment you probably can't imagine reaching five hundred miles – but you will and if you walk 500 miles you DESERVE a new pair of shoes!

If you have a lot of weight to lose, replace your shoes more frequently as you will be increasing pressure on the soles.

3. Get Used to wearing your Pedometer

Once you have your doctors approval and a comfortable pair of shoes, get used to wearing your pedometer and make sure you know how it works.

4. Establish Your Starting Point

Get yourself a notebook to use to monitor your progress and note down your starting data

Your current weight and measurements

Weigh yourself with no clothes before you step into the shower using a particular bathroom scale on a particular spot. This is so that it is easy to compare your weight in the same circumstances from one weighing session to the next. Many bathroom scales are inaccurate and vary depending where you weigh yourself but the exact weight doesn't really matter – just whether you are making pro-gress.

Add your chest, waist and hip measurements to your notebook as well as your upper arm and thigh circumference. Sometimes changes in measurement are more dramatic than changes to your weight especially if you are adding compact muscle and losing bulky fat tissue.

Your Average Daily Step Count

Every day for one week measure your step count and note it down in your notebook along with any physical exercise you take. Just go about your normal life wearing your pedometer and keep a note of your steps at the end of each day. It will be important as a starting reference so try not to skip this even if you are eager to get going.

Your Food Consumption

During the week keep a food diary. Note everything you eat over the week and especially take note of portion sizes. Don't feel guilty if you feel you are eating too much – just write down everything and then you will know where to begin your program.

If you are currently following another diet or weight loss program keep monitoring your calories/points etc as you normally would. If writing down everything seems boring, take a picture instead (a camera in your cell phone is handy for that). There's nothing like a set of pictures of your daily food intake to make you want to reduce it!

Your Clothing Choice

Select a piece of clothing which is now too tight for you so that you can use it as a measure of how well you are doing. Sometimes body weight can fluctuate for many reasons, and then clothing can help you see how much progress you are making.

5. Set Goals

What do you want to get out of this program?

I know that you want to lose weight otherwise you would have probably chosen another program but how will losing weight benefit you?

Do you want to

* fit into your old jeans or your best party dress
* look great at a wedding (maybe yours) or a party
* wear the clothes you want to wear
* get fit
* lower your blood pressure?

As well as setting a target weight, make your goals specific for what you really want and make them personal to you.

For example "I want to be fit enough to walk up the 3 flights of steps at work without needing to take a break half way up and I want to feel confident enough to wear my swimsuit on the beach without a cover-up."

Do You Need to Set A Time Limit on Your Goals?

Despite what all the goal setting manuals say I don't want you to set a time limit on achieving your aims for this walking with your pedometer program.

Why not?

The more pressure you put on yourself the worse you feel if you ever have a set-back and the less likely you are to make lifestyle changes which lead to **permanent** weight loss.

It is too easy to say I'm not going to make my target DATE so I may as well give up.

But you will always achieve a target weight and MAINTAIN it if you persevere and take things one step at a time (literally) on this program!

Even if you have a specific target date in mind such as your wedding you will always achieve more by thinking of your program as something you are doing for life and not for an event.

Let your wedding be motivation for keeping to your plan but don't set an end date after which you will give up walking and start eating for 6! You will simply end up putting all the weight back on again and quicker than you would have ever thought possible!

Write your goals in the notebook where you jotted down your weight, measurements etc.

By the way, don't be afraid to change your goals. As you become slimmer and fitter you will find yourself becoming more ambitious – you would not be the first person who decided they just wanted to be a bit fitter and then changed that to wanting to train to walk a marathon or go trekking along the Great Wall of China...

Target Weight

What weight should you set for your target?

It's important to be realistic for your height, bone structure and muscular make up. You probably know the kind of weight you are aiming for – the weight where you both look good and feel healthy – a weight which you don't have to go into starvation mode to maintain.

If you are in any doubt, about a healthy weight for you check out the latest government information online.

For example, this is a healthy weight chart from the food standards agency in the UK

http://www.eatwell.gov.uk/healthydiet/healthyweight/heightweightchart/

and the following link is from the US Center for Disease Control and Prevention which helps you compute where a healthy body mass index would lie (and tells you whether you are currently overweight)

http://www.cdc.gov/nccdphp/dnpa/healthyweight/assessing/bmi/index.htm

Remember that all **weight** is not equal – ten pounds of fat takes up an awful lot more space and therefore makes your body look a whole lot bigger than ten pounds of muscle.

With this program we are aiming to get smaller not just weigh less.

The emphasis on many diets is "lose weight at any cost" - and the cost is usually loss of muscle tissue, flabbiness and rapid weight gain where the lost muscle tissue is re-placed by fat – making you larger than ever!

Sense of Achievement Goals

If you have a lot to lose, then success can seem a long way off. Think about setting a goal for 5, 7 or 10lbs weight loss at a time and celebrate that success before moving on to set a new goal on the way to your ultimate target weight.

It's important that you not only monitor the RESULTS but also what you are doing to achieve them.

This program has built in sense of achievement goals which will help to motivate you – for example every day you meet your step and walking targets your confidence grows and you can feel good about yourself.

Continue to meet the daily achievement targets and you **WILL** achieve your other goals.

Your 28 Day Lose Weight With Your Pedometer Program

This plan contains three ways of achieving weight loss each and every day

1. A Daily Target

Setting yourself daily target for the number of steps you take during the course of the day

2. A Daily Walk

A main daily walk will contribute to your daily target and will also build up your aerobic fitness and muscles and turn your body into a fat-fighting machine

3. An Easy Way Of Reducing Calorie Consumption

You can choose any or all from 12 strategies for reducing calorie consumption without going hungry or giving up the foods you love.

Part 1: Your Daily Step Target

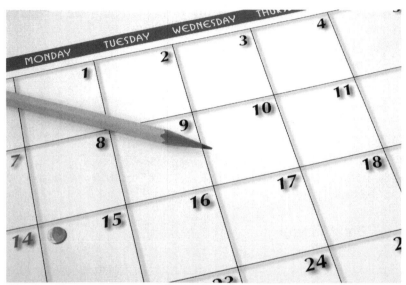

Start with average number of daily steps you took in your preparation week. (Add the total steps for the week and divide by the number of days) Round up the figure to the nearest 100.

So, for example, if you had the following results in your preparation week

Monday : 2456
Tuesday : 3987
Wednesday : 2109
Thursday : 4534
Friday : 4668
Saturday : 2460
Sunday : 3271

your total is 23,485 and your average (divide by 7) is 3355. You would then round up to 3,400.

In the first week add 2000 steps to your daily average to make your daily step target and then each week after that of the 4 week program add an additional 500 to your daily step goal. So week one in the above example you would aim for 5,400 daily steps, week two 5,900, week three 6,400 and week four 6,900.

Although a 2000 step increase may seem like quite a jump, it is actually pretty doable. In many cases you will achieve more than the required step increase simply by adding in your daily walk. You will need to make more effort to increase steps on those days when you do not take a longer walk.

How to Fit In More Steps

If you don't manage to get out walking on any day (and even those days you do) add more movement into your everyday life with the following ideas.

Use The Stairs

Take the stairs instead of the elevator whenever possible. Even if you can't climb to the 15th floor get off on the 12th or 13th floor and fit in more steps.

Make More Trips

When you have to take things upstairs or clear the table take as many trips as possible instead of trying to reduce them. Carry just a few things each time.

Walk While You Wait

When waiting for a train or plane walk the station or airport concourse rather than just standing or sitting waiting.

Walk and Chat

Arrange to meet a friend and go for a walk rather than spending half an hour on the phone.

Walk and Phone

If you do phone, use a cordless model and walk while you talk.

Walk Don't Email

Go and see a co-worker rather than sending an email.

Walk With Your Family

Suggest walking after dinner with your family – let them get some benefit too - and it's a great chance to chat away from the TV.

Walk With a Dog

Get a dog (or borrow one from a friend) and make sure it gets plenty of exercise.

Park Further Away

Park at least 100 yards away from wherever you want to go and don't take the car at all if you're only going a short distance.

Get Off the Bus Early

Get off the bus a stop or two before you need to and walk the rest of the way.

Tidy Up

Tidy your home, going in and out of each room to put things away as much as possible.

Take a Walking Break

Whenever you take a break at work, walk about a bit rather than just sitting. Use the kitchen and bathroom furthest away from your desk.

Walk and Browse

Try walking around while you're scanning a newspaper, catalog or magazine at home. Walk while you sort the junk mail.

Walk and View

Walk on a treadmill if you have one while watching TV or walk around during the commercial breaks

Find More Ways to Add Steps

Think about your own typical day, hour by hour, and the activities you do.

How could you get more steps with each one?

Could you be standing and moving at least some of the time rather than sitting?

One way to add a lot of steps in one fell swoop is with the daily walk we will be talking about in Part Two (see next page).

Monitor Your Daily Step Count

Each day note down your step total for the day in your notebook – so that you can see the progress you are making and give yourself a pat on the back each time you meet your daily target.

Part 2: Your Daily Walk

In order to get the aerobic and metabolic benefits of getting fitter and improve your fat burning potential, it's important, whenever you can, to include a longer walk in your day.

45 Minutes

The ideal is to **work up to** walking aerobically for at least 45 minutes every day at a speed of over 3.5 mph (after a 5 minute warm up at a comfortable pace).

During a 45 minute daily walk you will burn a whole heap of calories – many of them from fat. Here is an idea of the level of calories you can burn (based on a 150lb person).

Slow Pace: 2 mph

A 150lb person will burn 4 calories per minute and 180 in a 45 minute walk.

Medium Pace: 2.5 to 3 mph

The same person will burn 4.5 to 5 calories per minute and 210 to 240 in a 45 minute walk.

Brisk Pace: 3.5 to 4 mph

A walk at a brisk pace, would burn up 6 to 7 calories per minute and 270 to 315 on a 45 minute walk.

Fast Pace: 4.5 mph

Our 150lb walker would burn 8 calories a minute and proudly get rid of 375 calories over 45 minutes.

The idea is not that you burn as many calories as possible by going at a pace that is beyond you but that you sustain a pace as fast as you comfortably can for the period you are walking.

Of course, you can increase your pace as you get fitter to burn more calories and benefit more from the same amount of time you spend keeping fit and healthy.

Is 45 Minutes Tough To Fit In?

Now I know that 45 minutes walking a day is a tall order for many – where would you find that time? And you may not be at a level of fitness yet where you can easily manage this.

All I can say is that this is something to aim for.

If you can't manage a long walk every day then aim for 5 or even 3 days a week.

Whatever you can do is better than nothing but if you can manage to walk for 45 minutes on at least 3 days you will achieve valuable health and fitness benefits. (Any calories you use and steps you take always count towards your weight loss goals even if you can only do 5 minutes at a time but to get fit and maintain your fitness levels you need to work out regularly for longer periods).

You may think you are too busy to walk but you will often find that you come back so energized after your walk that you get twice as much done and often a walk will clear your head so that you can focus better on any issues you have too.

If your current level of fitness is the only thing holding you back then, don't worry, you can follow the plan here to build up your fitness and make good progress towards this aim in 28 days.

If you need to build up fitness before being able to do a long brisk walk then start with Fitness Plan A below. If you feel this is too easy for you move onto Fitness Plan B.

Walk at least 5 days each week to build up your fitness fast but if you can only manage 3 days then again that's great too! Go at your own pace – it's important that this becomes a part of your lifestyle rather than a burden.

Once you've completed Plan A you can move onto Plan B, to burn more calories and build up your level of fitness further before starting the 45 minute daily sessions.

Plan A To Build Up Your Level of Fitness

Week 1

On each of your walking days walk for **15 minutes** as follows

Walk at an easy pace for 5 minutes
Walk briskly for 5 minutes
Walk at an easy pace for 5 minutes

Week 2

On each of your walking days walk for **17 minutes** as follows

Walk at an easy pace for 5 minutes
Walk briskly for 7 minutes
Walk at an easy pace for 5 minutes

Week 3

On each of your walking days walk for **20 minutes** as follows

Walk at an easy pace for 5 minutes
Walk briskly for 10 minutes
Walk at an easy pace for 5 minutes

Week 4

On each of your walking days walk for **22 minutes** as follows

Walk at an easy pace for 5 minutes
Walk briskly for 12 minutes
Walk at an easy pace for 5 minutes

Plan B To Build Up Your Level of Fitness

Week 1

On each of your walking days walk for **25 minutes** as follows

Walk at an easy pace for 5 minutes
Walk briskly for 15 minutes
Walk at an easy pace for 5 minutes

Week 2

On each of your walking days walk for **30 minutes** as follows

Walk at an easy pace for 5 minutes
Walk briskly for 20 minutes
Walk at an easy pace for 5 minutes

Week 3

On each of your walking days walk for **30 minutes** as follows

Walk at an easy pace for 5 minutes
Walk as briskly as you can for 20 minutes. Try to increase the distance you cover with each of your workouts.
Walk at an easy pace for 5 minutes

Week 4

On each of your walking days walk for **30 minutes** as follows

Walk at an easy pace for 5 minutes
Walk as briskly as you can for 20 minutes. (Try and take in some more varied terrain without reducing your speed going up or increasing it going down. A 10% incline almost doubles the energy you use. Walking on rough ground or sand also increases your effort).
Walk at an easy pace for 5 minutes

Walking pace

You do have to walk a little faster than you normally would to burn maximum calories and increase your fitness.

People normally walk quite slowly. While a gentle stroll won't do you any harm it won't give you all the benefits you are seeking.

When you're supposed to be walking briskly, the easiest way to tell if you are working hard enough is to use the talk test. Walk fast enough so that you are a little breathless but can still talk – you can say your telephone number in one go but not your telephone number and your address! If your breathing is normal and you can shout out loud, sing or carry on a normal conversation you are not working hard enough. If you're finding it quite difficult to speak and can say only a couple of words at a time (or can't speak at all) the intensity is too high for the first few weeks – ease back until you are able to talk again.

If you like you can measure your level of effort with a heart rate monitor instead and aim for 60 – 70% of your maximum heart rate in the beginning. As you get fitter, you can push yourself a little harder – up to 80 or 85% of your maximum heart rate for full aerobic benefit.

If you're interested in measuring your speed, you can find out how fast you're walking by measuring out a mile in your car around your local area and timing yourself walking the distance at your usual brisk pace.

Before Each Walk

Have a Goal in Mind

Think about how far, how fast and how long you will walk and decide to achieve as much as you can without overdoing it.

Check the weather and wear suitable clothes

See the section on excuse avoidance if you think of the weather as an excuse! You may need hat, gloves, scarf and waterproof or sunscreen, sun hat, water bottle and sunglasses depending on the weather – just be sensible.

During Your Walk

Focus on the walk itself and enjoy it!

Always start out walking for 5 minutes at a slower pace than you will use during the main part of your walking session.

It's important to warm up so that your body has a chance to get ready for more vigorous exercise. Always keep your body warm during the warm up phase by wearing enough clothes – wear layers so that you can remove them if you become too hot later during the session. And you may need a hat and gloves when it's cold.

If you find walking a bit boring, and it is safe to do so, you can always listen to music, catch up on a podcast or enjoy an audio book. Or walk with a friend and catch up on their news (but see the section on who to walk with below)

After Your Walk

Make a note of how well you did, how you felt after your walk, how far and where you walked, how many steps you took and the distance (if you are measuring that) in your notebook.

You should see an improvement week after week, which will help you stay motivated.

Where to Walk

In the beginning convenience is so important because you have not got into the habit of walking and the benefits (though building up) are not as visible to you as they will be later on.

If you're going to walk regularly (and to lose weight you will need to), the easiest place to walk is to step outside your front door and walk around the block and back again – increasing the size of the "block" as you make progress. There's no need to make life complicated when you are just getting going.

You can also walk using your place of work as the starting point, either before or after work or during your lunch hour – same principle – walk around the block and back again.

Or walk your child to school and back if it's not too far for them – it's rarely the case unless you have a long way to go and your child is very small.

I heard of one mother who lost weight by walking while her child was doing after school activities – she walked from the football field or ballet studio around the block and back - an extra hour a few times a week when she would have normally been hanging around waiting.

If the weather is poor try walking around a local indoor shopping mall.

After a while the old familiar walks may get a bit boring but you will be feeling the benefits by then and will probably be willing to go a bit further afield.

At that point, liven up your walks by sometimes driving or getting the bus or train to different places.

You may like to stick with places close to home during the week and then venture further afield at the weekend.

When you want to add a bit of variety, try taking a walk around a different city or shopping mall. Find a river bank or beach. Or even just explore a different area of your town or city.

Personal Safety

Most of us will walk around day after day even after dusk and no harm will come our way – newspaper reports of muggings etc are news exactly because they are exceptional. I have personally walked for miles and miles by myself around my neighborhood without a care. But it makes sense to follow a few precautions to keep yourself as safe as possible...

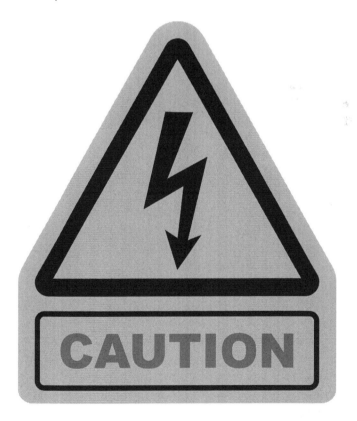

Tell Someone

Always tell someone where you are going and when you expect to be back or leave a note about where you are or message on your answering machine.

Carry ID

Carry ID with you and a note about any chronic medical condition.

Carry Your Cellphone

Take a mobile phone so you can easily contact someone if you get into difficulties especially if you are walking in a remote area

Don't Carry Valuables

Avoid wearing a lot of jewelry (which may look valuable even if it's not) and don't carry a lot of money

Think About A Personal Alarm

If you are worried, consider buying a personal alarm or whistle to keep with you to attract attention

Wear Bright Clothing

Wear reflective clothing if walking after dark and sensible clothing for the weather.

Make Sure You Can Hear

Avoid using a personal stereo if there are few people around so you can hear others approaching you – also avoid using headphones if it means you can't hear traffic when crossing roads etc

Get Confident

Build up your confidence with self defence classes – you're more likely to be a victim if you seem nervous or timid

Walk With A Friend

Walk with a companion if it makes you feel safer

Choose Your Route

Choose your route with care – you probably know the rough areas to avoid in your own area but if you're away from home ask the locals about safe places to walk and where to avoid

When to Walk

Any time is a good time to add a few steps with your pedometer so don't avoid walking on any occasion it makes sense to do so. But for your main walks, choose a time when you can get a good walking rhythm.

If possible, avoid the rush hour as your main walk if you walk in the city – it will be frustrating to continually stop and start due to crowds and traffic and you will be subject to more pollution than at other times.

If you are going mall-walking it makes sense to choose a quiet time such as when the shops have just opened so that you can walk unimpeded.

Who to walk with

I have to admit that, although I like walking with friends and family, I also like walking alone – it gives me a chance to think and clear the cobwebs. I can go at my own pace and set my own goals and I don't have to rely on anyone else to turn up – or get to a particular meeting place.

But I know that many people don't like the idea of solo walking.

If you can get a friend or family member to join you in following your walking program that's ideal – you will have fun walking together and the time will pass very quickly – just make sure you keep up the pace and don't get so engrossed in your conversation that you end up doing nothing but strolling!

If you don't know anyone already who could be your walking companion you could join a walking group. There may be day classes in your area which combine visiting places of interest with walking or you could join a group such as the Ramblers Association or local equivalent. It's a great way of meeting new friends while getting exercise.

The nearer to home the group, the more likely you are to get involved so make sure your group is not too far away.

A well-behaved dog who walks alongside you and is not constantly stopping and starting can be a real help in getting you out there and moving every day. You will both enjoy the exercise and companionship.

How to Walk - Walk this way to maximise the benefit

It may not have occurred to you that the way you walk can make walking harder work than it needs to be! But poor posture habits such as slumping, hunching your shoulders, not picking up your feet or holding your head down can all make walking less effective and more effort.

Walk Tall

Hold your head high and walk tall, letting your spine lengthen upwards. Look about 10 ft ahead, keeping your chin lifted. This keeps your neck and spine correctly aligned.

Relax Your Shoulders

Keep your shoulders loose and down – free from tension.

Swing Your Arms Naturally

Allow your arms to swing naturally and keep your hands loosely curled rather than clenched. For fitness walking where you want your arms to help you gain speed, hold your arms bent at about 90 degrees with your elbows close to your body. This allows your arms to swing faster than if they were extended and this will help you to walk more quickly. Move your arms forwards and backwards, not across your body and don't allow your hands to go higher than your shoulders.

Place Your Feet Correctly

The correct foot movement for walking is to land on your heel then roll through to the ball of your foot and push off with your toes.

Take Natural Strides

Take natural strides when walking fast. Take more steps rather than longer steps for a better workout.

Part 3: Adapt Your Eating Habits

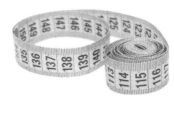

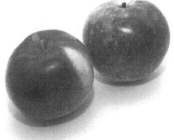

Provided you are not overeating (i.e. currently gaining weight) you can lose weight simply by taking more exercise. But I do not advise it.

Why Should You Change Your Eating habits as well as Walk?

You Will Lose Weight Faster

It is faster to lose weight by combining exercise with dietary changes and therefore more motivating – you will see progress more quickly

You Will Need Fewer Calories As You Lose Weight

As you lose weight it's a sad fact that you will need fewer calories to sustain your weight. You will either have to adapt your diet or do a lot more exercise (potentially more than you have time for) especially if you have a lot of weight to lose

You Need To Tackle The Real Issues

Food is often the main cause of a weight problem and therefore it has to be part of the solution too

You Will Get Back In Control

If you feel food is controlling your size and even your life it will help your confidence to get firmly back in control

You Don't Need to Go Hungry

There are painless changes you can make so you may as well make them

Remember how one of the preparations you made for your walking program entailed noting everything you ate for a week?

Now it's time to look at your food consumption.

First of all consider whether that amount of food causing you to

* maintain your current weight
* lose weight
* gradually gain weight?

What we are trying to achieve is a balance where:-

you eat slightly fewer calories than you need in a day

AND

you use up additional calories every day by increasing the amount of exercise (steps) you take.

If your current diet is helping you to lose weight

In this case, there is no need to change anything until your weight drops to a level where that is no longer the case – then you can simply follow the plan below.

On the other hand, you could begin making a few small changes in preparation for when you hit that point. (Remember as you lose weight you will need to eat fewer calories to continue losing).

The same holds true if you are following a diet or weight loss program which suits you – don't change what is working for you. The walking with your pedometer program works with any of the usual weight loss programs.

However, the main problem with commercial diets is that you usually go on them for a particular period of time – hopefully at least until you reach your target weight.

When they end, the tendency is to go back to your usual pattern of eating and exercise with the result that you gain all the weight back.

To avoid this problem, think about using the maintenance advice from your weight loss program as well as using some of the strategies in this guide and making them lifestyle changes. See also the "Plan for life" below.

If your current level of eating is simply maintaining your weight or making you gain weight

In this case, some changes are in order right away.

Here is a list of easy changes. There's nothing to dictate what you can and can't eat. There are no rules with this plan – you are an adult who can make your own decisions.

You simply choose the changes which are the easiest ones for you to put in place and live with. I advise taking one change at a time, working out how you can fit that change into your lifestyle with the least amount of fuss and making it a habit so that it stays with you forever.

That's the easiest way to make your weight loss permanent – make permanent lifestyle changes!

12 Easy changes

1. Reduce Quantities

Eat the same type of foods as you do now, but reduce your portion sizes.

If you don't put so much on your plate to start with and stop eating as soon as you are satisfied, you will naturally eat less.

Try not to cook too much or buy too much so that you are not tempted to eat more just to "save wasting food".

This first idea is the easiest to implement because you don't really have to change your habits to do that – you can still eat all your favourite foods – you just eat less of them.

If you are used to heaping your plate make gradual changes in the quantity you serve to give your stomach a chance to get used to smaller portions. If you reduce by a small amount each week your stomach will eventually shrink and not demand so much food.

2. Plan

By planning your food ahead of time (and cooking / preparing your snacks and meals in advance too wherever possible), you will not be tempted to nibble whatever is around while wondering what you will have for lunch or dinner.

Make all the calories you eat part of a meal or planned snack.

3. Stop Snacking After Dinner

Make dinner your final food of the day. Brush your teeth after dinner to draw a line under eating for the night. If you find it hard not to eat in the evenings while watching TV, take up another activity while you view – keep your hands busy with sewing or knitting or tackle the ironing pile. If you must have something to eat later on in the evening – make it a planned healthy snack rather than uncontrolled munching all evening.

4. Mindful Eating

Whenever you eat make it your sole activity – don't combine eating with reading, watching TV or preparing food. It's too easy not to notice how much you are consuming.

5. Eat More Vegetables and Salad

As an alternative to the first strategy (reducing the overall quantity of food but keeping the actual food the same) eat the same quantity of food but change the proportions of the various food types you serve – pile half your plate with vegetables and salad and leave only a quarter each for protein and carbohydrate.

6. Try New Foods

Experiment with cooking and serving something different more often. Choose 2 new healthy recipes every week and find your top 10 – the best recipes are those you enjoy immensely which also help you lose / maintain weight.

7. Avoid Drinking Calories

Calories in beverages add up but they don't fill you up, so avoid drinking calories – only eat them. Even foregoing one calorie-laden drink a day will have a big effect on your calorie count. The worst offenders are alcohol, milky drinks, fruit juices and fizzy soft drinks etc. Stick with water, tea and (non-milky) coffee as much as possible.

8. Know When To Eat and When to Stop

Eat only when you feel physically hungry and stop when you are satisfied rather than stuffed. Aim to leave the table feeling that you could comfortably eat something else (without being actually hungry) and give yourself a pat on the back when you don't overeat.

9. Allow Some Treats

Eat healthy food as much as possible but don't give up the junk you really love. Just keep the quantities moderate. Do give up those things you only eat "because they are there" - stop buying them altogether.

10. Don't Tempt Yourself

If you find it hard to resist eating certain things and can't stop eating them, then you may want to stop buying them for a while until you feel more in control.

11. Substitute Where It Doesn't Matter

Reduce the fat or calories in any food where it does not make a difference to you by making healthy substitutions. For example, remove the visible fat from meat and go for semi-skimmed rather than full fat milk. But don't reduce the enjoyment of your food when you do this. I believe you should get as much enjoyment out of it as possible by eating slowly and "savouring the flavour." It's often when we guzzle food without actually tasting it that we eat too much so it's important to enjoy your food and be aware what you are eating. If you LIKE substitutions as much as the real thing then feel free to go ahead. However, be careful you don't eat more because "they're low fat" or "they're only 100 calories".

12. Healthy Snacks

Snacking is one area where you can easily make a difference without having to go hungry.

Have healthy snacks readily available, include protein in your snacks and keep unhealthy snacks out of your house.

Think fruit, slices of tomato and cut up vegetables alongside a spoonful of peanut butter or a hard boiled egg. Or crackers spread thinly with low-fat cream cheese (provided you like the flavor of the low-fat version course!) or thin slices of hard cheese.

See Appendix 3 for more Healthy Snack Ideas.

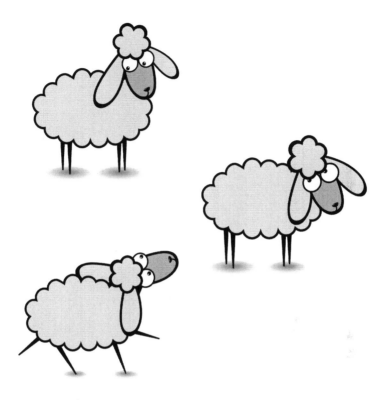

Above all else, **don't be a sheep**. You are an individual with your own food needs.

Just because someone else is eating or drinking something does not mean that you have to eat it too.

If you follow the crowd you're likely to become obese because that is what is happening in the general population these days.

What we see as a normal portion of food is often overeating especially if you eat out in restaurants.

Reset your idea of a normal eating and portions by listening to your body, eating when you are hungry and stopping when you have had just enough and no more.

Let the sheep roll away from the table feeling uncomfortable and loosening their waistbands. You don't have to be one of them.

Keep Track of Your Progress

As well as noting your daily steps and walks in your notebook, keep track of your food consumption. You can keep a food diary and calorie count if you like. Although I must admit I could never keep this up longer than a week or two – I know some of you like to do this.

What is particularly useful is if you keep notes of situations where you either were able to keep up your good eating habits or ones where you didn't.

In each case, think about and note down what strategy you used, what thoughts were going through your head and any ideas about what to do next time the same situation occurs to make things easier for yourself.

At the end of each week, take a note of your weight and try on your chosen piece of clothing to see how well you are doing. If you are not making as much progress as you hoped, examine your habits to see where you are going wrong. Are you still over-eating? What habits do you need to change?

Also remind yourself that you are probably not quite at the level where you are using many calories a day with your walking (especially if you are on one of the beginner plans or started with a low step count). The calories being burned and your weight loss will increase as you get fitter and increase your level of walking.

And then get right back on track. No one expects you to be perfect. You WILL succeed if you don't stop!

Plan for life

If you carry out the plan for 28 days you will become slim-mer, healthier and I hope you will have fun with it. Life is too short to follow a program you hate so this one is de-signed to become an enjoyable part of your life.

It is not meant to be one of those diet plans where you lose a massive amount of weight in 28 days and then put it all back on in a couple of weeks.

This one is meant to be with you forever so gradually wean yourself off bad habits and ease into exercise and you'll do just fine.

Maintenance Plan

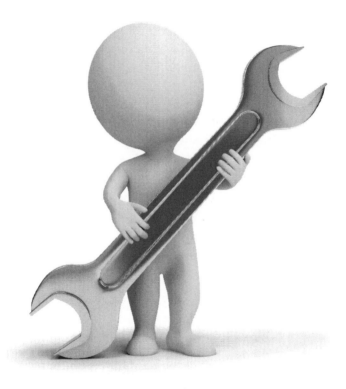

So how do you continue to lose weight or maintain the weight you lost after 28 days are up?

Part 1 : Daily Step Targets

The first thing to look at is how you are doing with your daily step counts.

Health authorities advise that we should be taking 10,000 steps every day so the best thing to do is to continue to increase your steps until you are at that level.

Maybe you are already there if you are taking daily walks. If not keep persevering with 500 extra steps a week until you reach the 10,000 level and then continue to walk at least 10,000 steps a day.

After a time you may find that you no longer need to wear your pedometer to judge how much exercise you are getting. You can leave it off for a while and just check out your average steps every now and again to ensure you're not deluding yourself :)

Part 2 : Daily Walks

If you continue walking at whatever level you've reached at the end of 28 days it will be hugely beneficial to you for the rest of your life.

However, if you want to continue to **improve** your fitness you do need to vary your workouts. The problem is that your body gets used to a particular exercise if all you do is repeat the same type of exercise at the same level over and over.

You can introduce more challenge in your walks by:-

Increasing the duration

Walking is not stressful on your joints so you can increase the length of your walk up to an hour or more

Picking Up The Pace

You will burn more calories and get fitter by walking faster – although there is a natural limit to this at which point you are jogging rather than walking!

Using Intervals

By introducing some speed bursts (or intervals) in your walking you will get fit and burn calories fast.

To do this, walk as fast as you can for a minute or two and then more slowly until you recover your breath and then fast again.

As your fitness improves you will find you can go flat out for longer (measured over distance or time) and will recover faster between bursts.

Varying The Terrain

Try some longer nature trails or hill-walks to increase the effort involved in your walk.

Adding Other Activities

Think about whether you want to move onto jogging or running or add variety to your fitness program by playing a sport on some days

Part 3 : Eating Habits

To help maintain your weight loss, keep up the new habits you have begun and make sure you don't creep back into your old ways. It's all too easy to slide back-wards especially if you don't keep an eye on things.

Continue to monitor how well you are doing - either by weighing yourself regularly and/or by using the "right-sized" clothing you selected.

If there are some habits you haven't adopted yet, add new good habits from the list until you reach your target weight.

Once you reach your target, it's important to nip any weight gain in the bud. If your weight ever creeps more than 2lbs over your target for more than a day or two, take action.

Reassess your habits and see if you have reintroduced any bad habits or reduced your level of exercise and get back on track. Two pounds is far easier to lose than ten!

Many people only take action once clothing starts to feel a bit tight but by this stage you have generally put on quite a few pounds so I find that it is best to use scales for weight maintenance.

You don't need to weigh yourself every day – once a week is about right.

With this plan in place and walking habits which are a permanent part of your lifestyle there will be no reason for you ever to pile on the pounds again after you lose them – you will be slimmer, fitter and healthier than you ever thought possible

Appendix 1:
Excuse Busters

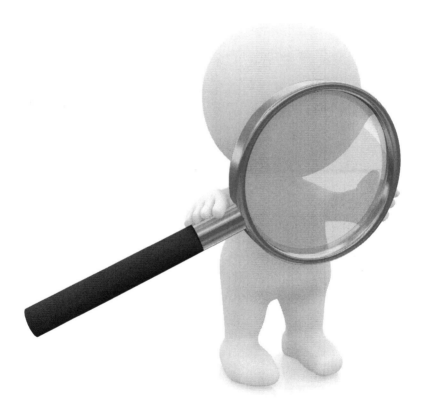

Don't Make the Weather an Excuse for not Walking

You can walk whatever the weather provided you have something to keep you dry when it's wet and warm when it's cold.

Many people start walking in spring and give up at the end of summer. But every part of the year has something to offer so enjoy the weather as it changes through the seasons.

Even if weather condition are so extreme it's not safe to walk outdoors, walk at the gym on a treadmill, walk around your home or try mall-walking where you walk around your local shopping centre.

So if it's not safe to walk due to icy paths and roads, you have alternatives. If it's too hot outside, walk early in the morning before the sun gets too warm or at dusk when it's little cooler or find a nice air-conditioned mall or gym. And if the weather man says stay home, then at the very least walk around your home.

Don't Make "No Time" an Excuse for not Walking

You probably have more time than you think – the problem is that our pockets of free time often come in disjointed parcels – 10 minutes here, an hour there.

You have to plan the time you will use for walking or it will just disappear. Block the time out in your schedule, make whatever arrangements you need to make and just do it.

If you find you mean to walk but life just gets in the way, then try to get your walking done first thing in the morning before anything else can interfere.

If you truly have no time at all then you have to prioritize and drop something. Are you really saying that your weight and your health is of so little importance to you that EVERY other activity you do takes precedence?

Don't Make "Too Much effort" an Excuse for not Walking

When you're worn out, it's surprising how much energy a walk in the fresh air can give you. Just say to yourself "I expect I'll feel better once I get out there", get out there and you WILL feel better!

Often one of the reasons why you feel sluggish is that you have not had enough exercise during the day, so if you feel tired in the evening walking will be a great re-viver.

Also make sure that you think of your walks as something positive you are doing for yourself not as a chore that needs to be done. This is "me" time when you have a chance to think and the opportunity to reduce stress and look after your body. You are caring for yourself in the best possible way.

Don't Make Caring for Children and Excuse for not Walking

Take them with you (no matter how much they moan it will do them good), book a babysitter or swap child care with another parent who likes to exercise.

If you have a small child to take along then this can be a help or a hindrance.

Walking with a pram or infant carrier is fine. When my eldest was born I walked miles and miles. I had a baby who did not sleep unless he was moving in a pram and I lost tons of pregnancy weight very quickly as a result.

Just be aware, walking with a pram may strain your lower back a bit so make sure you walk tall and don't lean forward too much (avoid sticking your bottom out).

With a small child out of the stroller yet not able to walk quickly or far you will have more of a challenge.

Take them out anyway – they will get fresh air and necessary exercise and you will build up more steps. If there's a play area where your child can safely play while you walk around the playground that's great. And you can have fun running after them – getting more steps all the while. If you haven't got enough steps or a decent workout from this kind of activity, go out for a longer walk yourself later on if you can.

Don't make Being Unfit or Suffering from a Health Condition an Excuse for not Walking

You can start the program at any level of fitness provided your doctor gives says it's Ok. If you can only walk 5 minutes, walk 5 minutes and build up gradually. You will be pleased you did.

Your doctor will also be able to tell you about exercise with your health condition – many health problems can be improved by walking.

Don't Make Boredom an Excuse for not Walking

If walking starts to get repetitive ring the changes with a bit of variety. Find different routes, walk with a friend, vary the intensity or simply listen to good music or a great audio book while you walk.

Don't Make Fear of the Dark an Excuse for Not walking

If you feel nervous about walking on your own at night carve out some time during the day to walk – for example, walk before work or during your lunch hour. Alternatively seek out populated places, walk in a mall which has evening opening hours or arrange to walk with a friend after dusk.

Now What's Your Excuse?

Appendix 2:
Your Questions
Answered

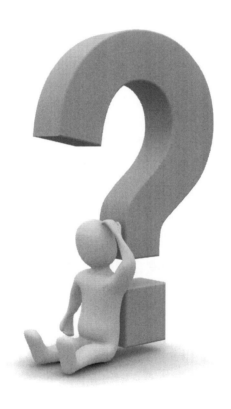

My pedometer doesn't tell me how many calories I am burning. How can I work this out?

Calculating how many calories you are burning can get quite complicated as it depends on a number of factors. The main ones are

a) how much you weigh (which affects how much effort your body is having to make)
b) how long you exercise for
c) how fast you go

As a rule of thumb, you could say that at a slow 2.5 mph pace you will burn roughly 2.1 calories per hour per pound of body weight.

At a medium 3.5 mph pace you would burn 2.4 calories per hour per pound of body weight.

And if you can achieve a 4.5 mph power walking pace, the figure jumps to 2.8 calories per hour per pound.

So if you weigh 200 lbs you will burn 420 calories (2.1 * 200) per hour at a slow pace, 480 calories (2.4 * 200) per hour at a medium pace and 560 calories (2.8 * 200) per hour at a fast pace.

The only sad thing about losing weight is that you burn fewer calories for the same time and pace. If you become half the size, you burn roughly half the calories, but it is still well worth losing weight, of course!

One way to counterbalance this reduction in calorie burning a little is to increase the proportion of lean tissue in your body (compared to the amount of fat) but you will inevitably do this if you take a lot of exercise rather than losing weight just by dieting. Lean tissue burns more calories than fat tissue even if you are only resting.

How Much Walking Is Too Much?

It really depends on your level of fitness. Although walk-ing can be a gentle exercise, it can also be quite punish-ing if you go fast and take to the hills.

It is always best to build up gradually and not to go mad from the very first day as that is when you find you are too sore to continue and get discouraged.

Try the programs in the book to build up your fitness if you are new to exercise.

And whatever level you are at, push yourself just a little more each day (in terms of effort or time or distance) to build up your fitness so that in the end, no walk is too much.

If you suffer any physical problems when you are walk-ing, have a check up with your doctor. It is probably only that you have pushed yourself too far for the stage of fit-ness you currently are, but it is better to be safe than sorry.

Do I Need to Take Any Other Exercise Other Than Walking?

Walking is good all round aerobic exercise and all you need for weight loss but for optimum health and all round fitness, you need to build your upper body strength with some form of weight or resistance training too. Core ex-ercises will help in flattening and tightening your tummy muscles as you lose weight and can help you stay lean and maintain good posture. Also, it is important to stay flexible as you get older and you would benefit from a program of regular stretching exercises or something like yoga too.

Do I Need To Stretch After Walking?

Stretching is always beneficial but it is not really essential to stretch every time you go out for a walk like you need to do if you go jogging or running. If you go power walking however some after workout stretches are useful to prevent soreness the next day.

If I Stop Walking Will I Get Fat Again?

It is a bit of an old wives' tale that when you stop exercising muscle turns to fat.

Muscles that you are no longer using so much will lose tone though and they will appear to be flabbier than they were.

Also if stopping your exercise program means that you are eating surplus calories again, those calories will turn into fat and you will eventually end up as large as you were before.

You just need to get the balance right between how much you are eating and the amount of exercise you are taking.

The problem is that as soon as you stop a positive habit by, for example, cutting back on walking it is easy for the pounds to creep on without you even noticing.

If you decide to change your exercise or eating habits once you reach your target weight, monitor very closely what is going on with your weight until you are sure that your current level of exercise and eating is Ok as a maintenance level.

You can do this by weighing yourself once a week and taking action if your weight ever creeps more than 2lbs above your target weight.

This way you avoid the sinking feeling of having to lose the same 10lbs over and over again.

2lbs is easy to lose with a little effort – 10lbs takes a lot more.

My goal is to get fit as well as lose weight. How can I make sure I am getting fitter as I walk?

You get fitter by exerting yourself just a little bit more every time you exercise and by pushing your body into the "training zone".

By getting a little bit breathless as you walk you know you are exerting yourself hard enough. You should still be able to hold a conversation however and if you have to keep stopping as you walk to catch your breath, you are pushing yourself too far.

If you want a foolproof way of detecting how hard you are working, use a heart rate monitor to detect when you are working in the "training zone" which is between 60% and 85% of your maximum heart rate (a figure that depends on your age and gender).

If you are new to fitness training you should train at the lower end of that range – around 60-65%. If you have been training for a few weeks you can aim for the middle of the range 70-75% and if you are very fit for the high end 80-85%.

As you get fitter you might find it difficult to build fitness just by walking on flat ground. You may need to incorporate some hills or stairs into your workout or start a running program. However for most of us getting to a level where we are able to walk at a power walking speed regularly will bring such enormous fitness benefits that we won't need to take this any further.

Am I Too Fat For This Program?

This walking program is for everyone who is able to walk, who wants to lose weight. It may be that you can only walk a very short distance at the start if you are very overweight but if you keep going and increase just a tiny bit each day your fitness will improve, and of course as your size reduces you will find exercise easier.

Back, foot, knee and ankle problems are very common problems that prevent those with a lot of excess weight from exercising.

If you find you can't walk due to problems like that you may need to take other forms of exercise that support your weight such as swimming or stationery cycling and make an effort with your diet to lose some excess pounds before you start your walking program.

Should I Walk Before or After Eating?

If you have not eaten for a long time, taking exercise can make you feel light headed, so it is best not to go walking when you are too hungry.

You can always munch on an apple as you walk – that is usually enough energy to keep you going without keeling over.

There is a tradition of taking a constitutional walk after dinner but make it a light meal (best for your weight loss efforts anyway) otherwise exercise may be uncomfortable.

Remember that there is no need to fuel up after exercise unless it is time for a meal (and definitely do not reward yourself with food) or you can end up negating any benefits by taking in more calories than you used up.

What is the best time of day to go walking?

Apart from being careful if you have had a heavy meal or need to eat (see above), any time that is convenient is a great time.

If the weather is hot, you will find it best to go early in the morning or after dusk, when it will be slightly cooler, but you could still walk at any time if you use an air conditioned mall for your walk!

There are a couple of reasons to get a longer walk in as early as possible though

a) in a polluted city, the air quality is usually best in the morning
b) if you are likely to have a busy day, taking your walk early gives you fewer chances to make excuses about not doing it and early success will set you up nicely for a positive day ahead.

I'd like to slim my legs. Will walking help? I'm worried that it will bulk up my muscles and make my thighs even chunkier

If you have weight to lose then this program will help you slim all over including your legs. It takes an awful lot of hard resistance exercise (especially in women) to add muscle bulk so your legs are more likely to slim than bulk up. If you would like to make sure that your muscles become more toned than bulky, then carry out a sequence of stretching exercises every day as well as walking to elongate the muscles.

How long will it take to lose 20lbs with this program? Can I lose weight faster by doing more?

There is no way to predict how quickly you will lose weight (because you should be tailoring the program to suit your level of fitness and eating habits and everyone is different) but if you follow all the guidelines you would typically lose around 1 to 2lbs a week.

If you want to calculate how much extra effort could help, a pound of fat is around 3500 calories so you would need to do a lot of walking to lose a single pound. As you will be adapting your eating habits as well if you follow the program, you don't need to do quite so much walking as you otherwise would.

Within reason, any extra walking you do or any extra effort you make with your diet will have an effect in helping you to lose weight faster.

If you go too mad with exercising and cutting back, however, you will force your body to go into starvation mode where it will try and preserve fat rather than burning it off. That's why the program advises moderate change and easing into exercise rather than drastic reduction in food and boot camp style effort.

In general, I have found the faster you lose weight, the faster you are likely to put it back on. A one to two pound weight loss a week that you create by making gradual lifestyle changes is the best way to lose weight and stay slim forever. If you have ever been on a radical diet where you lost a lot of weight, you will know how difficult it is to adjust to normal eating (and maintain your new weight) and you will understand the benefit of moderation.

Does this program work for everyone?

This program works for men, women, old, young – anyone who can walk and who needs to lose weight.

As long as your doctor says it is OK you can do it.

If you follow the program, you will lose weight. Simple!

I have never been able to stick to a weight loss program before. How can I make sure that I keep to this one?

Although this program gives guidelines for 28 days, it's better to see walking and eating healthily as a lifestyle change not as something that you do for 28 days and then give up.

The whole "being on a diet" idea of a period of deprivation, exercise and restraint followed by falling off the wagon, eating for a small country and not moving from your sofa is something to get away from for good if you want to stay slim and healthy for the rest of your life.

It's best to stick to the plan until you get the walking bug and feel good about your new eating habits and then it will become a natural part of your life - something you won't want to give up – especially when you see the effect your changes are having on your body.

Normal diets are a kind of enemy to struggle with. See this program as a friend who is helping you both look and feel good.

If you have a day where you eat too much or don't fit in as many steps as you wanted, don't beat yourself up about it.

One day like that doesn't stand a chance against all the days when you will be following good habits if you make the lifestyle changes recommended in this program.

How can I increase the effectiveness of my walk to lose weight faster?

The best thing you can do is to increase your speed. That way you burn more calories in the same amount of time.

You can have fun with this by measuring your time to complete a particular route you use on a regular basis and then try and beat your record each time you do it.

Also, try and walk for at least 45 minutes each time you go for a walk so that your body has a chance to get into the fat burning zone, rather than just using immediately available energy from the muscles.

Interval walking is also a particularly effective way to burn calories. This is where you alternate walking as fast as you can for a minute or two with a brisk pace for a minute or two until you recover for the period of your walk.

If you have countryside nearby, then walking on rough terrain (a soft sandy beach is great!) or in hills will certainly burn more calories too.

You might come across advice about wearing wrist or ankle weights. While it's true that if you wear weights, you will burn more calories when you cover the same distance, this can put an unnatural strain on your joints over a long walk and I would not advise that you do this.

It is better to walk unimpeded but faster!

Do I need to drink extra water when following a walking program?

It's important to stay hydrated, so, have a drink of water before you go for a walk and if you are going on a long walk (or if the weather is hot) take bottled water with you. Don't overdo it, as it's not that you need to drink extra gallons of water - you generally don't sweat when walking as much as you do with other forms of exercise.

****

If you have more questions, and you don't find the answers here, please get in touch using the contact form at walkoffweight,org and I will do my best to help.

Appendix 3:
Healthy Snack Ideas

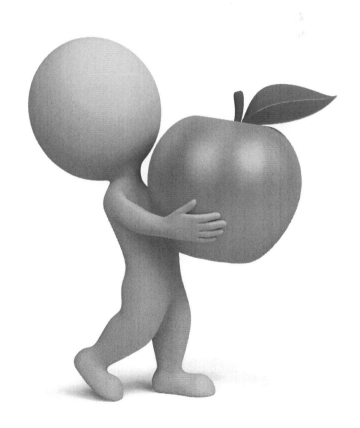

What To Do When The Munchies Strike

Sometimes you're in the mood for grazing all day and nothing will stop you. You just want to eat and you will hoover up anything you find.

When you know that this will happen sooner or later you're just tempting fate if your cupboards are filled with unhealthy snack foods and chocolate. It's as well to keep the junk out of the house completely.

And don't buy it just for the kids and/or your partner because you know it will end up in you as well as in them – and let's face it, they would be better off without it too!

If they have to have cake and cookies make sure you buy the stuff they like and you don't like so much - if anything like that exists :)

But even when you're eating normally, snacks are an essential part of a healthy diet. If you try to go too long without eating you'll find it harder to stick to eating modest portions of healthy food at mealtimes.

If you let yourself get too hungry, you'll end up just grabbing the quickest options you can find which as often as not will be fast food and takeaway.

So plan a couple of healthy snacks each day to keep you going. If you're not overeating at mealtimes you'll probably be hungry about 3 hours after eating – so this is probably mid-morning and mid-afternoon.

Also if you get into the situation where you come home absolutely starving and can't wait for dinner – have a quick healthy snack to take the edge off your appetite to allow yourself the time and energy to get a proper healthy meal together.

So, what can you eat as a healthy snack?

Here are 101 little snack ideas which are quick to pre-
pare, good to eat and won't break the calorie bank. Try
and vary the snacks you choose so they help you keep to
a good balanced diet and include some fruit and vegetable options so that you get lots of vitamins and minerals.

**Oh, and limit the ones with a (*) - they are not so
healthy but are just right when you need a treat**

A bowl of strawberries, with a spoonful of whipped cream
if you like

An oatcake or wholemeal cracker with a teaspoon of
crunchy, no-sugar-added peanut butter

A small bowl of no-sugar-added breakfast cereal and
skimmed milk

A single scoop of ice-cream (any kind) eaten very slowly
with a small spoon (*)

A sliced pear with a crumbling of blue cheese

A hard-boiled egg

6 almonds

A tall skinny latte

A juicy tomato cut into thin slices and topped with a few
torn basil leaves and a drizzle of one teaspoon of olive oil

Sticks of celery, cucumber, red and green (bell) peppers
and carrots dipped in a spoonful of any dressing

A small bowl of any soup

Two tablespoons of raisins (chocolate covered (*) if you
must!)

A small meringue nest filled with fresh fruit

A bowl of cherries

A small banana

Low fat natural yogurt with one teaspoon honey over chopped fruit

5-6 dried apricot halves

A large peach or nectarine

A slice of wholemeal toast with a teaspoon of preserves

Corn-on-the-cob with one teaspoon of butter or with with paprika or chilli powder

Small can of baked beans

Half a can of tuna in brine (drained) mixed with half can mixed beans

Half a ripe avocado eaten with a teaspoon

Two tablespoons pumpkin seeds

Handful of cherry tomatoes

Crispbread spread thinly with low fat cream cheese topped with cucumber and/or tomato slices

Small pot low fat cottage cheese with pineapple or any fruit

1 tablespoon low fat hummus and carrot sticks

A medium apple, sliced

2 satsumas

3 plums

2 squares of chocolate (*)

A bowl of mixed lettuce leaves, grated carrot, cucumber, tomato slices and tablespoon any dressing

Half a cantaloupe melon

2 kiwi fruit

Bowl of raspberries

A medium Orange

One thin crepe pancake with squeeze of lemon or orange juice and teaspoon of honey or sugar (*)

2 fresh apricots

2 rings fresh or canned pineapple

Lentil pate on low-fat cracker

Handful plain popcorn

One mango sliced

Bowl of blueberries

12 pretzel sticks

Half a grapefruit with a teaspoon of brown sugar sprinkle on the top and grilled (browned under the broiler)

1 rye-crispbread with teaspoon low-fat cream cheese and sliver of smoked salmon

Small scoop lemon sorbet

Small scoop frozen yogurt

1 sugar-free popsicle

Bowl any flavor jelly (Jell-O)

Freeze half a cup of any fruit juice to make a treat for hot weather

1 small slice wholemeal toast topped with half a mashed banana

Sugar free hot-chocolate made with skimmed milk or water (*)

Few dates

Celery stuffed with a little peanut butter or cream cheese

Rice cake with your favorite spread

Small glass red wine (*)

Half a pint of beer (*)

Half a cup of unsweetened apple sauce

2 bread sticks

1 or 2 tablespoons grated cheese on wholewheat toast, browned under the grill (broiler)

1 poached egg on wholemeal toast

Soda water on-the-rocks with a twist of lime or lemon, half and half with any pure fruit juice.

Creamy chive dip and raw vegetables (see recipe)

Frozen banana pieces. (Just place pieces of ripe banana on a tray in the freezer overnight.)

Tuna pate (see recipe) on wholewheat cracker

Slices of cucumber topped with small pieces of thinly sliced cheese or thinly spread with low fat cream cheese

Pizza cracker or two (see recipe)

Fill a pita pocket with lettuce, tomato, and a tablespoon of mixed bean salad – add a little dressing if needed.

Half a cup of cranberry juice over ice with club soda and an orange slice

A small slice of angel food cake (*)

2 boiled sweets (hard candy) (*)

Frozen grapes – just wash, dry and freeze separately overnight before bagging up.

Diced apple topped with low fat yogurt, a couple chopped nuts and cinnamon.

A fruit smoothie: Blend 1 cup skim milk or plain yogurt, a cup of diced fresh fruit, 2 teaspoons of honey and six large ice cubes until thick and smooth.

Slices of dill pickle

Raw mushroom caps

A handful of baked pita chips and salsa

2 crackers spread with mushroom pate (see recipe)

A slice of bruschetta (see recipe)

A scoop of strawberry and banana ice cream (see recipe)

Air-popped popcorn with a fresh lemon juice squeezed over it, and sprinkled with hot sauce (like Tabasco).

Fruit kebabs (kabobs) Just place pieeces of banana, melon, and grapes on bamboo skewers and pop them into the freezer on wax paper covered trays for a couple of hours for a cool treat.

A handful of roasted chickpeas (see recipe)

Combine a tablespoon orange marmalade, with a tablespoon orange liqueur. Drizzle over orange slices and top with a tablespoon of whipped cream.

A few kalamata olives

Frozen orange juice slush. Just add ice to orange juice and blend in the blender.

Toasted mixture of sunflower and pumpkin seeds

A scrambled egg cooked without oil in a non-stick pan on a thin slice of wholemeal toast or a piece of crispbread

Cheesy tomatoes (see recipe)

Blue cheese dip (see recipe) and crudites

Vegetable chips (see recipe)

Vegetable pate(see recipe) on crackers

Couple of slices of lean deli meat (cold cuts)

Chunks fresh coconut

A small glass of champagne(*)

2 fig bars

One slice of thin whole wheat toast spread with low fat cream cheese and topped with fresh fruit slices (such as peaches, banana slices, kiwi or strawberries) or you could use left-over roasted vegetables

One tortilla wrap (see recipe)

One handful of herby or cheesey baked tortilla chips (see recipe)

Recipes

Creamy chive dip

1 small tub or cup of cottage cheese
2 – 4 tablespoons milk
Chopped fresh chives to taste

Combine in a blender. Serve with raw vegetables.

Tuna Pate

Small tin of tuna in brine or water, drained
2 tablespoons plain yogurt
Chopped onion, celery and cucumber
¼ teaspoon dried mustard powder
Dash black pepper

Combine the ingredients and mix well.

Pizza crackers

Tomato slices or prepared tomato (pasta/pizza type)
sauce
Italian seasonings (herb mix)
Parmesan cheese
Crackers, bagel chips, crispbread, melba toast or pieces
pita bread

Place tomato slices or sauce on the cracker (or whatever
you are using). Sprinkle with Italian seasonings and a

little Parmesan. Place in a warm oven for a short time or grill (broil) until the cheese melts.

Mushroom Pate

40g (1.5 ounces) dried porcini mushrooms
100g (4 oz) chestnut mushrooms, sliced
1 garlic clove, chopped
100g (4oz) low fat cream cheese
2 teaspoons lemon juice
few drops Tabasco
freshly grated nutmeg

Soak the mushrooms according to the packet instructions (usually takes about 30 minutes). Spray a pan with oil and stir fry the chesnut mushrooms with the garlic for a minute. Add the drained soaked mushrooms and fry until the mixture is dry. Put the cheese, lemon juice, mushrooms in a processor and process until smooth. Add black pepper, Tabasco and nutmeg to taste. Chill in the fridge. Remove from fridge 30 minutes before serving.

Bruschetta

1 small French loaf
1 clove garlic
Good quality olive oil spray
25g (1oz) fresh basil leaves, chopped
4 ripe plum tomatoes, chopped or small tin chopped tomatoes, juice drained off

Cut the bread in diagonal slices and toast on both sides until golden and crisp under the grill or broiler. Rub the hot toast all over on each side with the raw garlic and spray with a little of the olive oil spray. Mix the tomatoes with the basil leaves and divide among the slices – serve immediately.

Strawberry and Banana ice-cream

2 cups strawberries, fresh or frozen, unsweetened
1 medium banana, cut into chunks
1 ½ cups yogurt, low fat, plain
2 tablespoons strawberry preserves, reduced-sugar type

Blend all the ingredients in a blender until smooth. Either use an ice cream machine to freeze or pop into a plastic freezer container and freeze for 1 ½ hours. Transfer mixture into a large bowl and beat with electric mixer until light and fluffy. Return to the container and freeze for another 30 minutes. Beat again in bowl and serve immediately or keep in the freezer covered for up to 2 weeks.

Roasted chickpeas

3 cups home cooked chickpeas
1 tablespoon olive oil
salt

Drain chickpeas and while still warm mix with the the oil and a little salt. Place in a single layer on a baking tray and roast in a hot oven (220 degrees centigrade/425 F/Gas Mark 7) until brown (about 20 minutes)

Cheesey tomatoes (for 1 or 2)

1 large beefsteak tomato
25 - 50g (1 - 2oz) reduced-fat cheese, such as cheddar
or Monterey Jack, thinly sliced
A few crisp lettuce leaves
Triangles wholewheat toast

Pre-heat the grill or broiler. Slice the tomato thickly and place on flat ovenproof dish or grill pan. Cover with the slices with the thinly sliced cheese and grill until golden and bubbly. Serve on top of lettuce leaves and with a couple of toast triangles.

Blue cheese dip

225g (8oz) cottage cheese
50g (2oz) blue cheese
1 tablespoon milk, cream or soured cream

Process all the ingredients together in a blender until smooth. Use as dip or salad dressing. A little goes a long way!

Vegetable "fries"

1 medium carrot
1 medium potato
1 medium sweet potato
1 tablespoon olive oil.

Cut into shapes like chunky fries. Boil for 4 minutes to soften. Drain and return to the warm pan. Add the olive oil and combine well. Bake in a hot (200 degrees centigrade/ 400 F/ Gas Mark 6) pre-heated oven for about 40 minutes until brown and tender

Vegetable pate

1 onion, sliced
2 garlic cloves
125g (4 oz) chopped carrots
125g (4 oz) chopped swede (or turnip)
1 teaspoon grated orange zest
half teaspoon ground coriander (cilantro)
2 tablespoons low fat cream cheese

freshly grated nutmeg and pepper to taste

Cook the vegetables and garlic in just enough boiling water to cover until soft and most of the water has evaporated off. Drain and process with the coriander, zest and cheese in a blender. Add nutmeg and pepper to taste. Chill for an hour before serving.

Tortilla wrap

One 4 or 5 inch tortilla
1 teaspoon low-fat mayonnaise mixed with 1 teaspoon low-fat soured cream
Grated/shredded vegetables – e.g. mixture carrot, courgette (zucchini), red (bell) pepper, cucumber, salad onions)
2 tablespoons grated cheese

Spread the tortilla with the mayonnaise mixture. Top with the vegetables and then the grated cheese and wrap.

Herby/cheesey tortilla chips

Flour or corn tortillas
Parmesan or dried mixed herbs

Spray light coating oil on flour or corn tortilla. Lightly sprinkle with the Parmesan or dried mixed herbs. Cut into 8 wedges. Bake in a hot oven (200 degrees centigrade/ 400 F/ Gas Mark 6) for about 8 minutes or until crispy.

About The Author

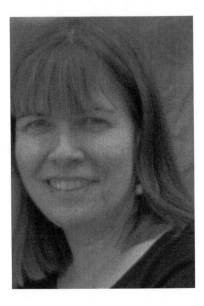

Author Jan Small is a weight loss coach and health and beauty writer. She believes that every woman is beautiful in her own way and that we can all be even more beautiful if we look after ourselves – there's no need to spend an arm and a leg on expensive products – it's more about attention to detail and making the effort to look good.

As far as weight loss goes, Jan believes it's important to keep things both simple and enjoyable so that it is easy to stick to the principles of whatever program you are following for life.

There is nothing more dispiriting than losing weight and then gaining it all back in much less time than it took you to lose, so it's important to make changes that you don't mind being a permanent part of your lifestyle.

You might not be as strict with yourself but at least you are not going to rebel against your whole program and end up back at square one – or worse – weighing even more than before.

Jan says

"I can be as lazy as the next person when it comes to keeping fit. I've tried to take up running a few times over the years but always ended up with sore joints and I had to give up after a few weeks every time.

That means walking is right up my street and it's my main way of keeping fit now along with yoga for strength and toning.

I don't use my pedometer all the time these days but if the pounds are starting to creep on, out it comes and I use it for an almost instant weight loss fix along with paying a bit more attention to what I'm eating"

You can find more of Jan's writing at the following places online

Beauty Top To Toe:
http://beautytoptotoe.com

Weight Loss Motivation:
http://weight-loss-motivation-program.com

Walk Off Weight:
http://walkoffweight.org

Follow Jan on Twitter:
http://twitter.com/beautytoptotoe/

Printed in Great Britain
by Amazon.co.uk, Ltd.,
Marston Gate.

12262713R00060